The Ultimate Gui
Meal Preparation

Quick and Easy Recipes for Busy People to Get Back in Shape
and Lose Weight

Lola Rogers

© Copyright 2021 - All rights reserved.

The content contained within this book may not be reproduced, duplicated or transmitted without direct written permission from the author or the publisher.

Under no circumstances will any blame or legal responsibility be held against the publisher, or author, for any damages, reparation, or monetary loss due to the information contained within this book. Either directly or indirectly.

Legal Notice:

This book is copyright protected. This book is only for personal use. You cannot amend, distribute, sell, use, quote or paraphrase any part, or the content within this book, without the consent of the author or publisher.

Disclaimer Notice:

Please note the information contained within this document is for educational and entertainment purposes only. All effort has been executed to present accurate, up to date, and reliable, complete information. No warranties of any kind are declared or implied. Readers acknowledge that the author is not engaging in the rendering of legal, financial, medical or professional advice. The content within this book has been derived from various sources. Please consult a licensed professional before attempting any techniques outlined in this book.

By reading this document, the reader agrees that under no circumstances is the author responsible for any losses, direct or indirect, which are incurred as a result of the use of information contained within this document, including, but not limited to, — errors, omissions, or inaccuracies.

Table of contents

Limey Savory Pie 6

Supreme Raspberry Chocolate Bombs 10

The Perfect Orange Ponzu 12

Hearty Cashew and Almond butter 16

The Refreshing Nutter 18

Elegant Cranberry Muffins 20

Refreshing Mango and Pear Smoothie 23

Epic Pineapple Juice 26

Choco Lovers Strawberry Shake 28

Healthy Coffee Smoothie 31

Blackberry and Apple Smoothie 33

Almond Buttery Green Cabbage 36

Mesmerizing Brussels and Pistachios 38

Brussels's Fever 41

Hearty Garlic and Kale Platter 43

Acorn Squash with Mango Chutney 45

Roasted Herb Crackers 47

Banana Steel Oats 50

Swiss Chard Omelet 52

Hearty Pineapple Oatmeal 55

Traditional Frittata 57

Pepperoni Omelet 60

Eggy Tomato Scramble 62

Breakfast Fruit Pizzas 64

Peanut Butter Overnight Oats 66

Sporty Baby Carrots 68

Saucy Garlic Greens 70

Garden Salad 72

Spicy Cabbage Dish 75

Yogurt with Walnuts & Honey 77

Simple Caprese Sandwich 79

Cottage Cheese Honey Toast 80

Pimento Cheese Sandwich 82

Tomato Salad 84

Exuberant Sweet Potatoes 86

Ethiopian Cabbage Delight 88

Spice Trade Beans and Bulgur 90

Tofu Chow Mein 93

BOW TIES WITH SAUSAGE & ASPARAGUS 95
PORK AND BALSAMIC STRAWBERRY SALAD 97
PEPPERED TUNA KABOBS 100
WEEKNIGHT CHICKEN CHOP SUEY 102
CUCUMBER AND ZUCCHINI SOUP 105
CROCKPOT PUMPKIN SOUP 107

Limey Savory Pie

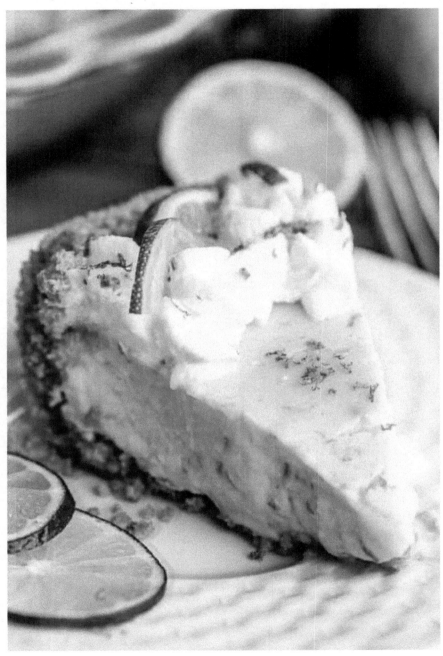

Serving: 12

Prep Time: 5 minutes

Cooking Time: 5 minutes

Freeze Time: 2 hours

Ingredients:

- 1 tablespoon ground cinnamon
- 3 tablespoons almond butter
- 1 cup almond flour

For the filling:

- 3 tablespoons grass-fed almond butter
- 4 ounces full-fat cream cheese
- ¼ cup coconut oil
- 2 limes
- A handful of baby spinach Stevia to taste

How To:

1.   Mix cinnamon and almond butter to form a crumble mixture.

2.   Press this mixture into the bottom of 12 muffin cups.

3.   Bake for 7 minutes at 350 degrees F.

4.   Juice the lime and grate for zest while the crust is baking.

5.   Take a food processor and add all the filling ingredients.

6.   Blend until smooth.

7.   Let it cool naturally.

8.   Pour the mixture in the center.

9.   Freeze until set and serve.

Nutrition (Per Serving)

Total Carbs: 2g

Fiber: 1g

Protein: 3g

Fat: 1g

Supreme Raspberry Chocolate Bombs

Serving: 6

Prep Time: 10 minutes

Cooking Time: 10 minutes

Freeze Time: 1-hour

Ingredients:

- ½ cacao almond butter
- ½ coconut manna
- 4 tablespoons powdered coconut almond milk
- 3 tablespoons granulated stevia
- ¼ cup dried and crushed raspberries, frozen

How To:

1. Prepare your double boiler to medium heat and melt the cacao almond butter and coconut manna.

2.   Stir in vanilla extract.

3.   Take another dish and add coconut powder and sugar substitute.

4.   Stir the coconut mix into the cacao almond butter, 1 tablespoon at a time, making sure to keep mixing after each addition.

5.   Add the crushed dried raspberries.

6.   Mix well and portion it out into muffin tins.

7.   Chill for 60 minutes and enjoy!

Nutrition (Per Serving)

Total Carbs: 7g

Fiber: 1g

Protein: 11g

Fat: 21g

The Perfect Orange Ponzu

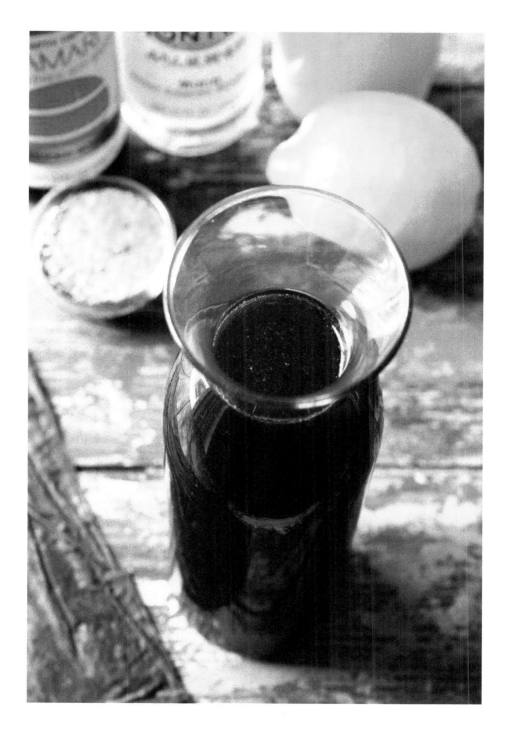

Serving: 8

Prep Time: 30 minutes

Cook Time: 5 minutes

Ingredients:

- ¼ cup coconut aminos
- ½ cup rice vinegar
- 2 tablespoons dry fish flakes
- 1 (1 inch) square kombu (kelp)
- 1 orange, quartered

How To:

1. Take a saucepan and place it over medium heat.

2. Add coconut aminos, rice vinegar, fish flakes, kombu, orange quarters and let the mixture sit for 30 minutes.

3. Bring the mix to a boil and immediately remove from the heat.

4.   Let it cool and strain through a cheesecloth.

5.   Serve and enjoy!

Nutrition (Per Serving)

Calories: 15

Fat: 0g

Carbohydrates: 4g

Protein: 0.8g

Hearty Cashew and Almond butter

Serving: 1 and ½ cups

Prep Time: 5 minutes

Cook Time: Nil

Ingredients:

- 1 cup almonds, blanched
- 1/3 cup cashew nuts
- 2 tablespoons coconut oil
- Sunflower seeds as needed
- ½ teaspoon cinnamon

How To:

1. Pre-heat your oven to 350 degrees F.

2. Bake almonds and cashews for 12 minutes.

3.   Let them cool.

4.   Transfer to food processor and add remaining ingredients.

5.   Add oil and keep blending until smooth.

6.   Serve and enjoy! Nutrition (Per Serving)

Calories: 205

Fat: 19g

Carbohydrates: g[MOU3]

Protein: 2.8g

The Refreshing Nutter

Serving: 1

Prep Time: 10 minutes

Ingredients:

- 1 tablespoon chia seeds
- 2 cups water
- 1 ounces Macadamia Nuts
- 1-2 packets Stevia, optional
- 1 ounce hazelnut

How To:

1.   Add all the listed ingredients to a blender.

2.   Blend on high until smooth and creamy.

3.   Enjoy your smoothie.

Nutrition (Per Serving)

Calories: 452

Fat: 43g

Carbohydrates: 15g

Protein: 9g

Elegant Cranberry Muffins

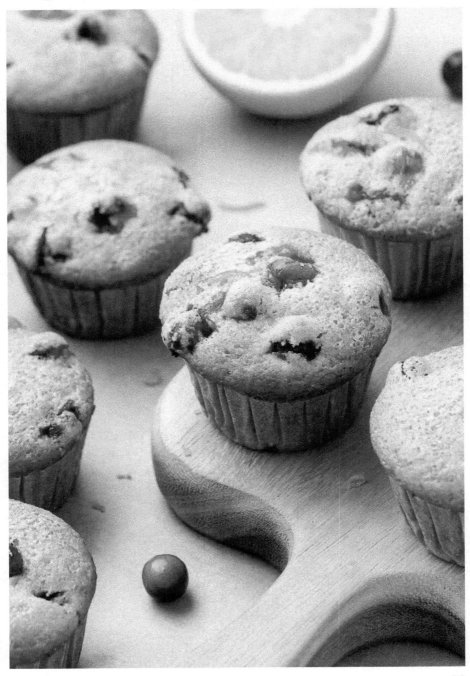

Serving: 24 muffins

Prep Time: 10 minutes

Cooking Time: 20 minutes

Ingredients:

- 2 cups almond flour
- 2 teaspoons baking soda
- ¼ cup avocado oil
- 1 whole egg
- ¾ cup almond milk
- ½ cup Erythritol
- ½ cup apple sauce
- Zest of 1 orange
- 2 teaspoons ground cinnamon
- 2 cup fresh cranberries

How To:

1.   Pre-heat your oven to 350 degrees F.

2.   Line muffin tin with paper muffin cups and keep them on the side.

3.   Add flour, baking soda and keep it on the side.

4.   Take another bowl and whisk in remaining ingredients and add flour, mix well.

5.   Pour batter into prepared muffin tin and bake for 20 minutes.

6.   Once done, let it cool for 10 minutes.

7.   Serve and enjoy!

Nutrition (Per Serving)

Total Carbs: 7g

Fiber: 2g

Protein: 2.3g

Fat: 7g

Refreshing Mango and Pear Smoothie

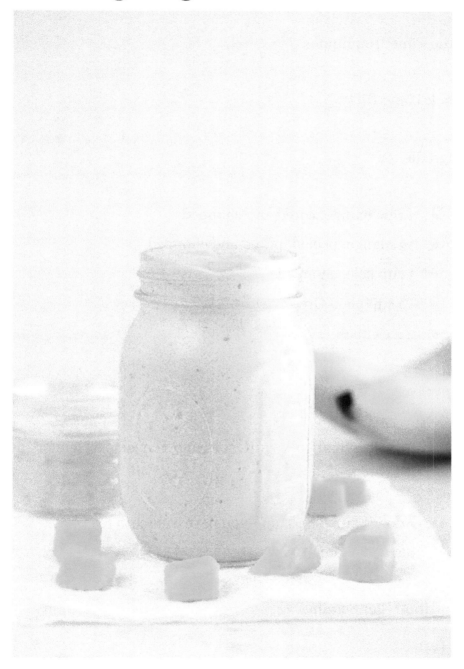

Serving: 1

Prep Time: 10 minutes

Cook Time: Nil

Ingredients:

- 1 ripe mango, cored and chopped
- ½ mango, peeled, pitted and chopped
- 1 cup kale, chopped
- ½ cup plain Greek yogurt
- 2 ice cubes

How To:

1.   Add pear, mango, yogurt, kale, and mango to a blender and puree.

2.   Add ice and blend until you have a smooth texture.
3.   Serve and enjoy!

Nutrition (Per Serving)

Calories: 293

Fat: 8g

Carbohydrates: 53g

Protein: 8g

Epic Pineapple Juice

Serving: 4

Prep Time: 10 minutes

Cook Time: nil

Ingredients:

- 4 cups fresh pineapple, chopped
- 1 pinch sunflower seeds
- 1 ½ cups water

How To:

1.   Add the listed ingredients to your blender and blend well until you have a smoothie-like texture.

2.   Chill and serve.

3.   Enjoy!

Nutrition (Per Serving)

Calories: 82

Fat: 0.2g

Carbohydrates: 21g

Protein: 21

Choco Lovers Strawberry Shake

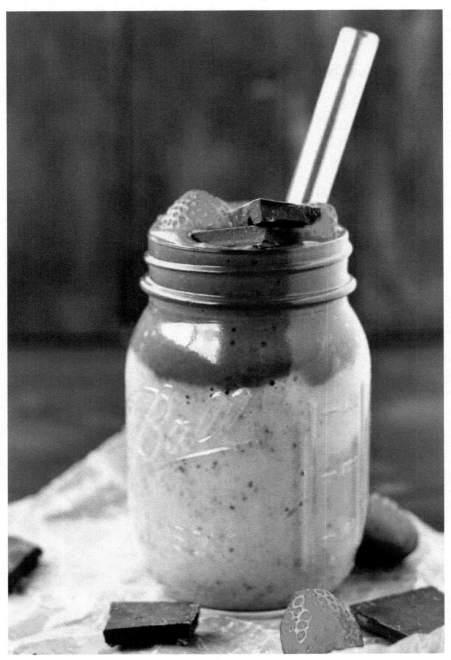

Serving: 1

Prep Time: 10 minutes

Ingredients:

- ½ cup heavy cream, liquid
- 1 tablespoon cocoa powder
- 1 pack stevia
- ½ cup strawberry, sliced
- 1 tablespoon coconut flakes, unsweetened
- 1 ½ cups water

How To:

1.   Add listed ingredients to blender.

2.   Blend until you have a smooth and creamy texture.

3.   Serve chilled and enjoy!

Nutrition (Per Serving)
Calories: 470

Fat: 46g

Carbohydrates: 15g

Protein: 4g

Healthy Coffee Smoothie

Serving: 1

Prep Time: 10 minutes

Ingredients:

- 1 tablespoon chia seeds
- 2 cups strongly brewed coffee, chilled
- 1-ounce Macadamia Nuts
- 1-2 packets stevia, optional
- 1 tablespoon MCT oil

How To:

1. Add all the listed ingredients to a blender.

2. Blend on high until smooth and creamy.
3. Enjoy your smoothie.

Nutrition (Per Serving)

Calories: 395

Fat: 39g

Carbohydrates: 11g

Protein: 5.2g

Blackberry and Apple Smoothie

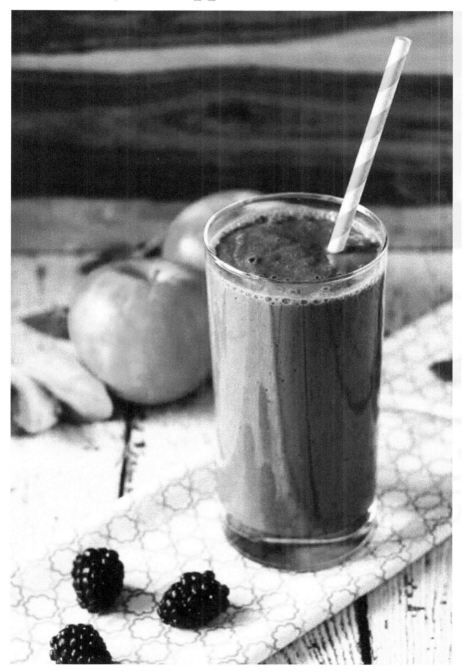

Serving: 2

Prep Time: 5 minutes

Ingredients:

- 2 cups frozen blackberries
- ½ cup apple cider
- 1 apple, cubed
- 2/3 cup non-fat lemon yogurt

How To:

1.   Add the listed ingredients to your blender and blend until smooth.

2.   Serve chilled!

Nutrition (Per Serving)

Calories: 200

Fat: 10g

Carbohydrates: 14g

Protein 2g

Almond Buttery Green Cabbage

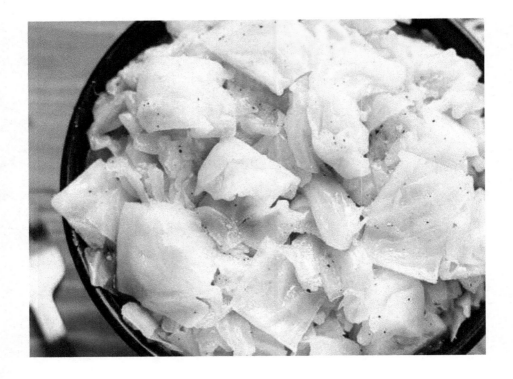

Serving: 4

Prep Time: 10 minutes

Cook Time: 15 minutes

Ingredients:

- 1 ½ pounds shredded green cabbage

- 3 ounces almond butter
- Sunflower seeds and pepper to taste
- 1 dollop, whipped cream

How To:

1. Take a large skillet and place it over medium heat.

2. Add almond butter and melt.
3. Stir in cabbage and sauté for 15 minutes.
4. Season accordingly.
5. Serve with a dollop of cream.
6. Enjoy!

Nutrition (Per Serving)

Calories: 199

Fat: 17g

Carbohydrates: 10g

Protein: 3g

Mesmerizing Brussels and Pistachios

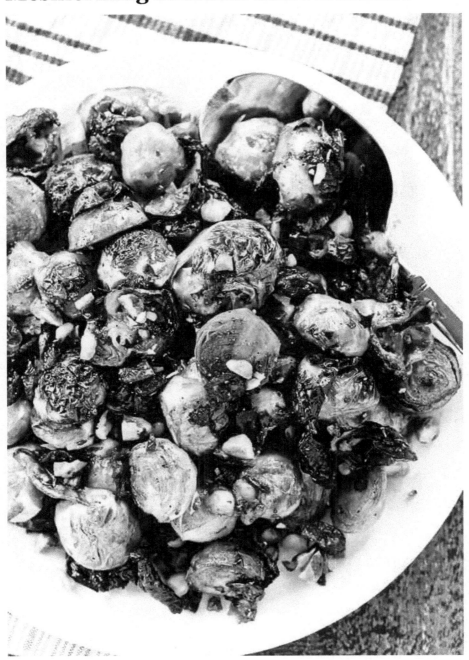

Serving: 4

Prep Time: 15 minutes

Cook Time: 15 minutes

Ingredients:

- 1-pound Brussels sprouts, tough bottom trimmed and halved lengthwise
- 1 tablespoon extra-virgin olive oil
- Sunflower seeds and pepper as needed
- ½ cup roasted pistachios, chopped
- Juice of ½ lemon

How To:

1.   Pre-heat your oven to 400 degrees F.

2.   Line a baking sheet with aluminum foil and keep it on the side.

3.   Take a large bowl and add Brussels sprouts with olive oil and coat well.

4.   Season sea sunflower seeds, pepper, spread veggies evenly on sheet.

5.   Bake for 15 minutes until lightly caramelized.

6.   Remove from oven and transfer to a serving bowl.

7.   Toss with pistachios and lemon juice.

8.   Serve warm and enjoy!

Nutrition (Per Serving)

Calories: 126

Fat: 7g

Carbohydrates: 14g

Protein: 6g

Brussels's Fever

Serving: 4

Prep Time: 10 minutes

Cook Time: 20 minutes

Ingredients:

- 2 tablespoons olive oil
- 1 yellow onion, chopped
- 2 pounds Brussels sprouts, trimmed and halved
- 4 cups vegetable stock
- ¼ cup coconut cream

How To:

1. Take a pot and place it over medium heat.

2. Add oil and let it heat up.
3. Add onion and stir-cook for 3 minutes.
4. Add Brussels sprouts and stir, cook for 2 minutes.
5. Add stock and black pepper, stir and bring to a simmer.

6. Cook for 20 minutes more.

7. Use an immersion blender to make the soup creamy.

8. Add coconut cream and stir well.

9. Ladle into soup bowls and serve.

10. Enjoy!

Nutrition (Per Serving)

Calories: 200

Fat: 11g

Carbohydrates: 6g

Protein: 11g

Hearty Garlic and Kale Platter

Serving: 4

Prep Time: 5 minutes

Cook Time: 10 minutes

Ingredients:

- 1 bunch kale
- 2 tablespoons olive oil
- 4 garlic cloves, minced

How To:

1.   Carefully tear the kale into bite sized portions, making sure to remove the stem.

2.   Discard the stems.

3.   Take a large sized pot and place it over medium heat.

4.   Add olive oil and let the oil heat up.

5.   Add garlic and stir for 2 minutes.

6. Add kale and cook for 5-10 minutes.

7. Serve!

Nutrition (Per Serving)

Calories: 121

Fat: 8g

Carbohydrates: 5g

Protein: 4g

Acorn Squash with Mango Chutney

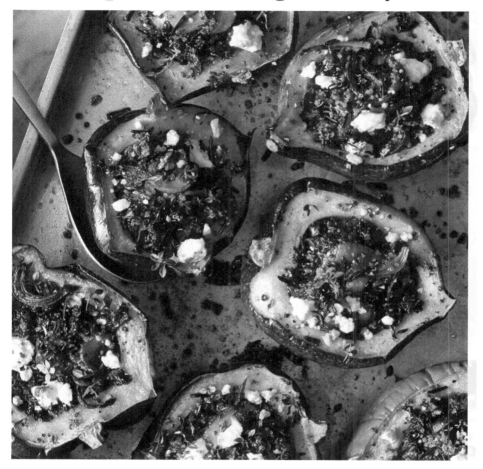

Serving: 4

Prep Time: 10 minutes

Cook Time: 3 hours 10 minutes

Ingredients:

- 1 large acorn squash
- ¼ cup mango chutney
- ¼ cup flaked coconut
- Salt and pepper as needed

How To:

1.   Cut the squash into quarters and remove the seeds, discard the pulp.

2.   Spray your cooker with olive oil.

3.   Transfer the squash to the Slow Cooker and place lid.

4.   Take a bowl and add coconut and chutney, mix well and divide the mixture into the center of the Squash.

5.   Season well.

6.   Place lid on top and cook on LOW for 2-3 hours.

7. Enjoy !

Nutrition (Per Serving)

Calories: 226

Fat: 6g

Carbohydrates: 24g

Protein: 17g

Roasted Herb Crackers

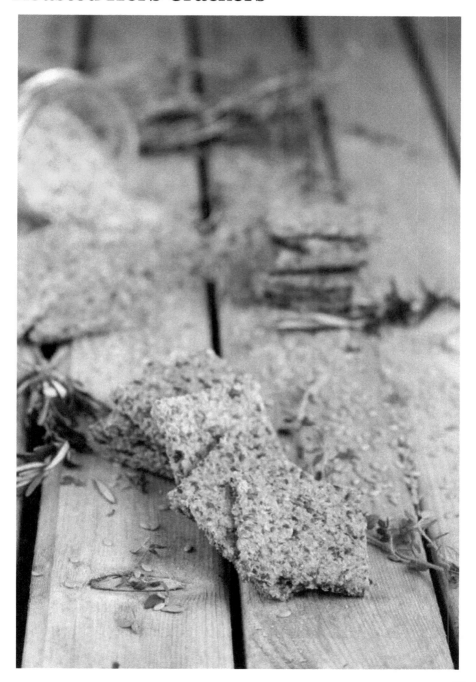

Serving: 75 Crackers

Prep Time: 10 minutes

Cook Time: 120 minutes

Ingredients:

- ¼ cup avocado oil
- 10 celery sticks
- 1 sprig fresh rosemary, stem discarded
- 2 sprigs fresh thyme, stems discarded
- 2 tablespoons apple cider vinegar
- 1 teaspoon Himalayan sunflower seeds
- 3 cups ground flaxseeds

How To:

1. Preheat your oven to 225 degrees F.

2. Line a baking sheet with parchment paper and keep it on the side.

3. Add oil, herbs, celery, vinegar, sunflower seeds to a kitchen appliance and pulse until you've got a good mixture.

4. Add flax and puree.

5.   Let it sit for 2-3 minutes.

6.   Transfer batter to your prepared baking sheet and spread evenly, dig cracker shapes.

7.   Bake for hour , flip and bake for hour more.

8.   Enjoy!

Nutrition (Per Serving)

Calories: 34

Fat: 5g

Carbohydrates: 1g

Protein: 1.3g

Banana Steel Oats

Serving: 3

Prep Time: 10 minutes

Cook Time: 15 minutes

Ingredients:

- 1 small banana
- 1 cup almond milk
- ¼ teaspoon cinnamon, ground
- ½ cup rolled oats
- 1 tablespoon honey

How To:

1.   Take a saucepan and add half the banana, whisk in almond milk, ground cinnamon.

2.   Season with sunflower seeds.

3.   Stir until the banana is mashed well, bring the mixture to a boil and stir in oats.

4.   Reduce heat to medium-low and simmer for 5-7 minutes until the oats are tender.

5.   Dice the remaining half banana and placed on the highest of the oatmeal.

6.   Enjoy!

Nutrition (Per Serving)

Calories: 358

Fat: 6g

Carbohydrates: 76g

Protein: 7g

Swiss Chard Omelet

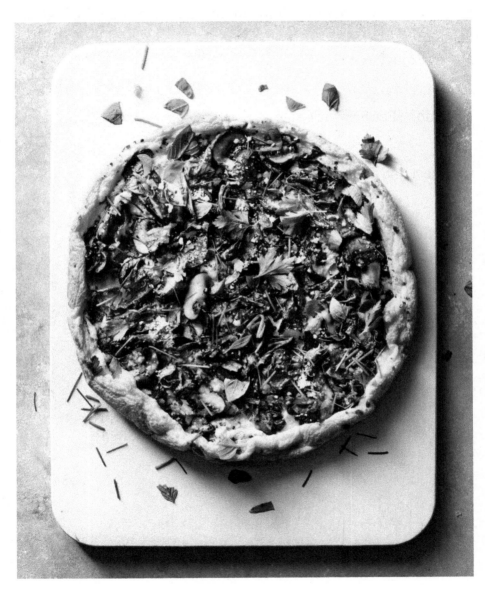

Serving: 2

Prep Time: 5 minutes

Cook Time: 5 minutes

Ingredients:

- 2 eggs, lightly beaten
- 2 cups Swiss chard, sliced
- 1 tablespoon almond butter
- ½ teaspoon sunflower seeds
- Fresh pepper

How To:

1.   Take a non-stick frypan and place it over medium-low heat.

2.   Once the almond butter melts, add Swiss chard and stir-cook for two minutes.

3.   Pour the eggs into the pan and gently stir them into Swiss chard.

4.   Season with garlic sunflower seeds and pepper.

5.   Cook for two minutes.

6.   Serve and enjoy!

Nutrition (Per Serving)

Calories: 260

Fat: 21g

Carbohydrates: 4g

Protein: 14g

Hearty Pineapple Oatmeal

Serving: 5

Prep Time: 10 minutes

Cook Time: 4-8 hours

Ingredients:

- 1 cup steel-cut oats
- 4 cups unsweetened almond milk
- 2 medium apples, sliced
- 1 teaspoon coconut oil
- 1 teaspoon cinnamon
- ¼ teaspoon nutmeg
- 2 tablespoons maple syrup, unsweetened
- A drizzle of lemon juice

How To:

1.   Add listed ingredients to a pan and blend well.

2.   Cook on very low flame for 8 hours/or on high flame for 4 hours.

3.   Gently stir.

4.   Add your required toppings.

5.   Serve and enjoy!

6.   Store within the fridge for later use; confirm to feature a splash of almond milk after re-heating for added flavor.

Nutrition (Per Serving)

Calories: 180

Fat: 5g

Carbohydrates: 31g

Protein: 5g

Traditional Frittata

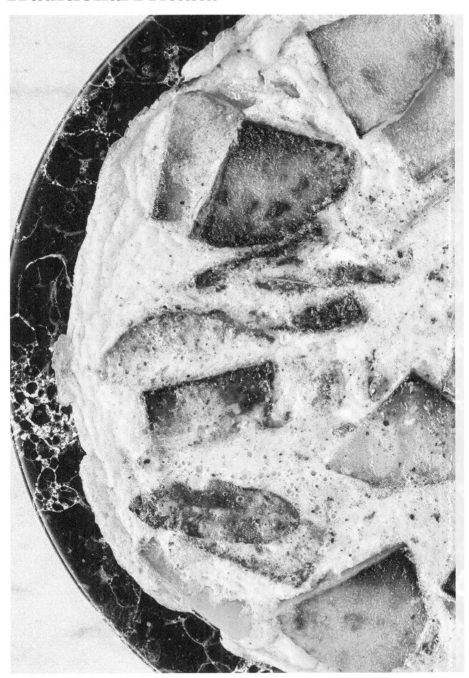

Serving: 6

Prep Time: 10 minutes

Cook Time: 5 minutes

Ingredients:

- 2 tablespoons almond milk
- Just a pinch pepper
- 6 eggs, cracked and whisked
- 2 tablespoons parsley, chopped
- 1 tablespoon low-fat cheese, shredded
- 1 cup of water

How To:

1.   Take a bowl and add the eggs, almond milk, pepper, cheese, and parsley. Whisk well.

2.   Take a pan that might slot in your Instant Pot and grease with cooking spray.

3.   Pour the egg mix into the pan.

4.   Add a cup of water to your pot and place a steamer basket.

5.   Add the pan within the basket.

6.   Lock the lid and cook on high for five minutes.

7.   Release the pressure naturally over 10 minutes.

8.   Remove the lid and divide the frittata amongst serving plates.

9.   Enjoy!

Nutrition (Per Serving)

Calories: 200

Fat: 4g

Carbohydrates: 17g

Protein: 6g

Pepperoni Omelet

Serving: 2

Prep Time: 5 minutes

Cook Time: 20 minutes

Ingredients:

- 3 eggs
- 7 pepperoni slices
- 1 teaspoon coconut cream
- Salt and freshly ground black pepper, to taste
- 1 tablespoon butter

How To:

1.   Take a bowl and whisk eggs with all the remaining ingredients in it.

2.   Then take a skillet and warmth butter.

3.   Pour quarter of the egg mixture into your skillet.

4.   After that, cook for two minutes per side.

5.   Repeat to use the whole batter.

6.   Serve warm and enjoy!

Nutrition (Per Serving)

Calories: 141

Fat: 11.5g

Carbohydrates: 0.6g

Protein: 8.9g

Eggy Tomato Scramble

Serving: 2

Prep Time: 10 minutes

Cook Time: 5 minutes

Ingredients:

- 2 whole eggs
- ½ cup fresh basil, chopped
- 2 tablespoons olive oil
- ½ teaspoon red pepper flakes, crushed
- 1 cup grape tomatoes, chopped
- Salt and pepper to taste

How To:

1.   Take a bowl and whisk in eggs, salt, pepper, red pepper flakes and blend well.

2.   Add tomatoes, basil, and mix.

3. Take a skillet and place over medium-high heat.

4. Add the egg mixture and cook for five minutes until cooked and scrambled.

5. Enjoy!

Nutrition (Per Serving)

Calories: 130

Fat: 10g

Carbohydrates: 8g

Protein: 1.8g

Breakfast Fruit Pizzas

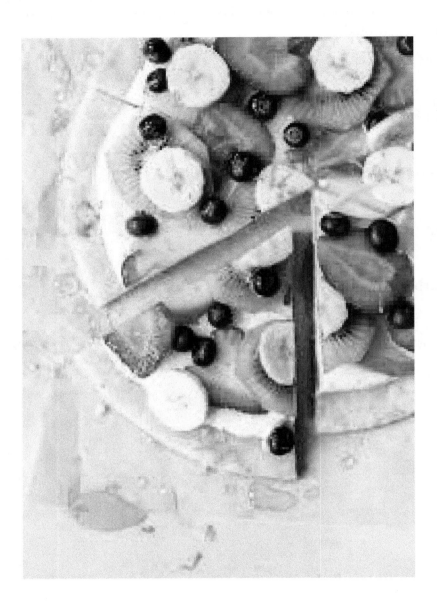

Ingredients

- Two whole-wheat pita flatbreads
- 7 ounces Arla Original Cream Cheese
- 1-2 teaspoons honey
- 1/2 teaspoon pure vanilla extract
- Three kiwi skin removed and sliced
- 1/2 cup sliced strawberries
- 1/2 cup blackberries
- 1/4 cup blueberries
- Two raspberries for the center

Instructions

1.   Preheat the oven to broil. Put the entire wheat pita flatbreads within the oven. Broil for 1 minute and switch over. Broilfor one minute more. you'll also toast the entire pita bread during a kitchen appliance . Set the dough aside to chill.

2.   Take a bowl and blend the cheese , honey, and vanilla. Spread the cheese on the pita bread.

3.   Decorate the fruit on top of the cheese . dig slices and serve immediately.

4.   Note-you can use your favorite fruit. Bananas, peaches, pineapple, oranges, nectarines would even be good!

Peanut Butter Overnight Oats

Ingredients

- Oats

- Half of cup unsweetened plain almond milk (or sub other dairy-free milk, such as coconut, soy, or hemp!)
- 3/4 Tbsp of chia seed
- 2 Tbsp of natural salted peanut butter or almond butter (creamy or crunchy // or sub other nut or seed butter)
- 1 Tbsp of maple syrup (or sub coconut sugar, natural brown sugar, or stevia to taste) half of cup gluten-loose rolled oats (rolled oats are best, vs. Steel-cut or quick-cooking)
- Toppings optional
- Sliced banana, strawberries, or raspberries
- Flaxseed meal or additional chia seed
- Granola

Instructions

1.   Take alittle bowl with a lid, add almond milk, chia seeds, spread , and syrup (or every othersweetener) and stir with a

spoon to mix . The spread doesn't got to be alright blended with the almond milk (doing so leaves swirls of spread to enjoy the next day).

2.   Add oats and stir a couple of extra times. Then depress with a spoon to form sure all oats were moistened and areimmersed in almond milk.

3.   Cover tightly with a lid or seal and set within the fridge overnight (or for a minimum of 6 hours) to place/soak.

4.   the next day, open and knowledge as is or garnish with preferred toppings.

5.   Overnight oats will preserve within the refrigerator for 2-three days, though high-quality within the primary 12-24 hours in our experience. Not freezer friendly.

Nutrition

Calories: 452, Fat: 22.8g, Saturatedfat: 4.1g, Sodium: 229mgPotassium:

479mgCarbohydrates: 51.7g Fiber: 8.3gSugar: 15.8g Protein: 14.6g

Sporty Baby Carrots

Serving: 4

Prep Time: 5 minutes

Cook Time: 5 minutes

Ingredients:

- 1-pound baby carrots
- 1 cup water
- 1 tablespoon clarified ghee
- 1 tablespoon chopped up fresh mint leaves
- Sea flavored vinegar as needed

How To:

1.   Place a steamer rack on top of your pot and add the carrots.

2.   Add water .

3.   Lock the lid and cook at high for two minutes.

4.   Do a fast release.

5.   Pass the carrots through a strainer and drain them.

6.   Wipe the insert clean.

7.   Return the insert to the pot and set the pot to Sauté mode.

8.   Add drawn butter and permit it to melt.

9.   Add mint and sauté for 30 seconds.

10.   Add carrots to the insert and sauté well.

11.   Remove them and sprinkle with little bit of flavored vinegar on top.

12.   Enjoy!

Nutrition (Per Serving)

Calories: 131

Fat: 10g

Carbohydrates: 11g

Protein: 1g

Saucy Garlic Greens

Serving: 4

Prep Time: 5 minutes

Cook Time: 20 minutes

Ingredients:

- 1 bunch of leafy greens Sauce
- ½ cup cashews soaked in water for 10 minutes
- ¼ cup water
- 1 tablespoon lemon juice
- 1 teaspoon coconut aminos
- 1 clove peeled whole clove
- 1/8 teaspoon of flavored vinegar

How To:

1.   Make the sauce by draining and discarding the soaking water from your cashews and add the cashews to a blender.

2.   Add water , juice , flavored vinegar, coconut aminos, garlic.

3.   Blitz until you've got a smooth cream and transfer to bowl.

4.   Add ½ cup of water to the pot.

5.   Place the steamer basket to the pot and add the greens within the basket.

6.   Lock the lid and steam for 1 minute.

7.   Quick-release the pressure.

8.   Transfer the steamed greens to strainer and extract excess water.

9.   Place the greens into a bowl .

10.   Add lemon aioli and toss.

11.   Enjoy!

Nutrition (Per Serving)

Calories: 77

Fat: 5g

Carbohydrates: 0g

Protein: 2g

Garden Salad

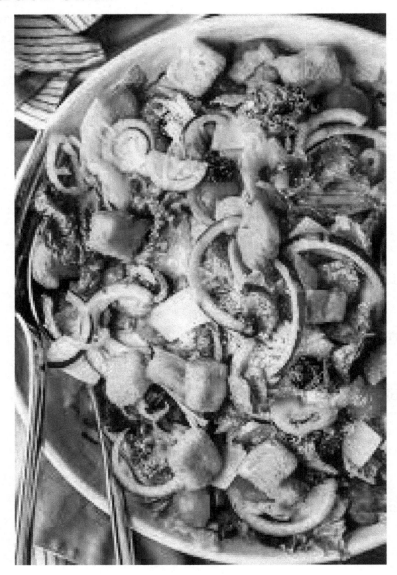

Serving: 6

Prep Time: 5 minutes

Cook Time: 20 minutes

Ingredients:

- 1 pound raw peanuts in shell
- 1 bay leaf
- 2 medium-sized chopped up tomatoes
- ½ cup diced up green pepper
- ½ cup diced up sweet onion
- ¼ cup finely diced hot pepper
- ¼ cup diced up celery
- 2 tablespoons olive oil
- ¾ teaspoon flavored vinegar
- ¼ teaspoon freshly ground black pepper

How To:

1. Boil your peanuts for 1 minute and rinse them.
2. The skin are going to be soft, so discard the skin.
3. Add 2 cups of water to the moment Pot.
4. Add herb and peanuts.
5. Lock the lid and cook on high for 20 minutes.
6. Drain the water.

7.   Take an outsized bowl and add the peanuts, diced up vegetables.

8.   Whisk in vegetable oil , juice , pepper in another bowl.

9.   Pour the mixture over the salad and blend .

10.   Enjoy!

Nutrition (Per Serving)

Calories: 140

Fat: 4g

Carbohydrates: 24g

Protein: 5g

Spicy Cabbage Dish

Serving: 4

Prep Time: 10 minutes

Cooking Time: 4 hours

Ingredients:

- 2 yellow onions, chopped
- 10 cups red cabbage, shredded
- 1 cup plums, pitted and chopped
- 1 teaspoon cinnamon powder
- 1 garlic clove, minced
- 1 teaspoon cumin seeds
- ¼ teaspoon cloves, ground
- 2 tablespoons red wine vinegar
- 1 teaspoon coriander seeds
- ½ cup water

How To:

1.   Add cabbage, onion, plums, garlic, cumin, cinnamon, cloves, vinegar, coriander and water to your Slow Cooker.

2. Stir well.

3. Place lid and cook on LOW for 4 hours.

4. Divide between serving platters.

5. Enjoy!

Nutrition (Per Serving)

Calories: 197

Fat: 1g

Carbohydrates: 14g

Protein: 3g

Yogurt with Walnuts & Honey

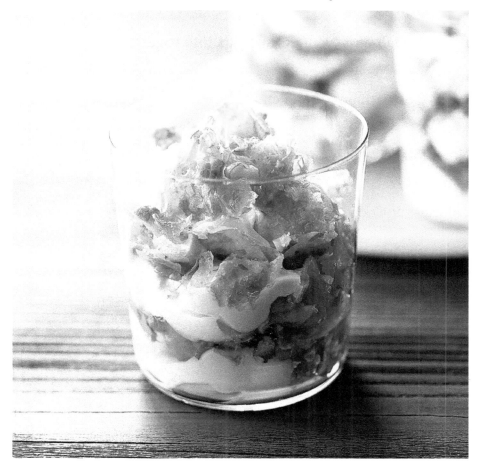

Ingredients

- Walnuts-Nuts, black, dried-1/4 cup, chopped-31.3 grams
- Non-fat greek yoghurt-Nonfat, plain-480cup-480 grams
- Honey-2 tsp-14.1 gram

Directions

1.   Rough-chop walnuts and mix into yogurt.

2.   Top with honey and enjoy!

Nutrition

Calories520Carbs32gFat20gProtein56gFiber2gNet

carbs30gSodium174mgCholesterol24mg

Simple Caprese Sandwich

Ingredients

- Sourdough bread, French or Vienna, Two slices, 192 grams
- Mozzarella cheese
- Whole milk 2 oz 56.7 grams
- Tomatoes - Red, ripe, raw, year-round average
- Four slices, medium (1/4" thick)

Instructions

Cut a large slice of sourdough in half (or use two small slices). Top one slice with 1oz of sliced mozzarella and then two slices of tomatoes. The flavor is mild, so season with salt pepper if desired.

Nutrition

Calories707Carbs104gFat17gProtein34gFiber5gNet

carbs99gSodium1515mgCholesterol45mg

Cottage Cheese Honey Toast

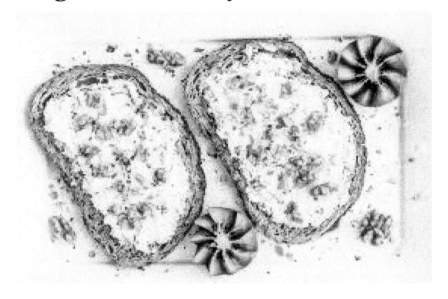

Ingredients

- Whole-wheat bread-Commercially prepared-
- Two slice-56 grams

Cottage cheese- 1% milkfat-1 cup, (not packed)-226 grams

Honey-2 tbsp-42 grams

Directions

Toast bread to your liking. Spread with cottage cheese and drizzle with honey. Enjoy!

Nutrition

Calories432Carbs65gFat4gProtein35gFiber3gNet

carbs61gSodium1174mgCholesterol9mg

Pimento Cheese Sandwich

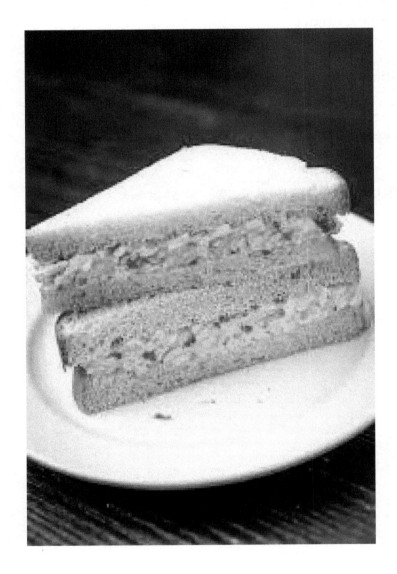

Ingredients

- Pimento cheese-Pasteurized process-2 oz-56.7 grams

- Multi-grain bread-Four slices regular-104 grams

Directions

1.	Spread the pimento cheese on each side of bread.

And then on the other slice of bread to form a sandwich. Enjoy!

Nutrition

Calories488Carbs46gFat22gProtein26gFiber8gNet

carbs38gSodium915mgCholesterol53mg

Tomato Salad

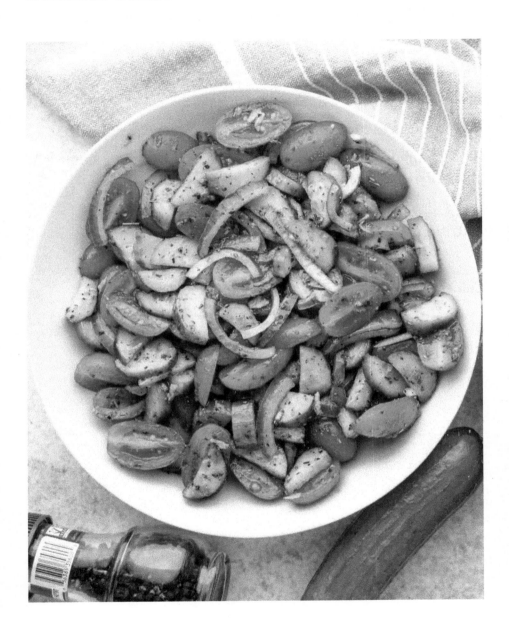

Ingredients

- Vinegar-Cider-2 2/3 tbsp-39.4 grams
- Cucumber-Peeled, raw-Two medium-402 grams
- Onions-Raw-1/2 large-75 grams
- Tomatoes-Red, ripe, fresh, year-round average
- Three medium whole (2-3/5" dia)-369 grams
- Water-Plain, clean water-1/2 cup-118 grams

Directions

Peel and slice cucumbers into coins. Cut tomatoes into pieces. Dice red onion. Add vinegar and water and mix well.

Nutrition

Calories153Carbs31gFat1gProtein6gFiber9gNet

carbs22gSodium32mgCholesterol0mg

Exuberant Sweet Potatoes

Serving: 4

Prep Time: 5 minutes

Cook Time: 7-8 hours

Ingredients:

- 6 sweet potatoes, washed and dried

How To:

1.   Loosely botch 7-8 pieces of aluminium foil within the bottom of your Slow Cooker, covering about half the area .

2.   Prick each potato 6-8 times employing a fork.

3.   Wrap each potato with foil and seal them.

4.   Place wrapped potatoes within the cooker on top of the foil bed.

5.   Place lid and cook on LOW for 7-8 hours.

6.   Use tongs to get rid of the potatoes and unwrap them.

7.   Serve and enjoy!

Nutrition (Per Serving)

Calories: 129

Fat: 0g

Carbohydrates: 30g

Protein: 2g

Ethiopian Cabbage Delight

Serving: 6

Prep Time: 15 minutes

Cook Time: 6- 8 hours

Ingredients:

- ½ cup water
- 1 head green cabbage, cored and chopped
- 1-pound sweet potatoes, peeled and chopped
- 3 carrots, peeled and chopped
- 1 onion, sliced
- 1 teaspoon extra virgin olive oil
- ½ teaspoon ground turmeric
- ½ teaspoon ground cumin
- ¼ teaspoon ground ginger

How To:

1.   Add water to your Slow Cooker.

2.   Take a medium bowl and add cabbage, carrots, sweet potatoes, onion and blend .

3.   Add vegetable oil , turmeric, ginger, cumin and toss until the veggies are fully coated.

4.   Transfer veggie mix to your Slow Cooker.

5.   Cover and cook on LOW for 6-8 hours.

6.   Serve and enjoy!

Nutrition (Per Serving)

Calories: 155

Fat: 2g

Carbohydrates: 35g

Protein: 4g

Spice Trade Beans and Bulgur

Total Time

Prep: 30 min. Cook: 3-1/2 hours

Makes

10 servings

Ingredients:

- 3 tablespoons canola oil, isolated
- 2 medium onions, slashed
- 1 medium sweet red pepper, slashed
- 5 garlic cloves, minced
- 1 tablespoon ground cumin
- 1 tablespoon paprika
- 2 teaspoons ground ginger
- 1 teaspoon pepper
- 1/2 teaspoon ground cinnamon
- 1/2 teaspoon cayenne pepper
- 1-1/2 cups bulgur

- 1 can (28 ounces) squashed tomatoes

- 1 can (14-1/2 ounces) diced tomatoes, undrained

- 1 container (32 ounces) vegetable juices

- 2 tablespoons darker sugar

- 2 tablespoons soy sauce

- 1 can (15 ounces) garbanzo beans or chickpeas, flushed and depleted

- 1/2 cup brilliant raisins

- Minced crisp cilantro, discretionary

Directions:

1.   In an enormous skillet, heat 2 tablespoons oil over medium-high warmth. Include onions and pepper; cook and mix until delicate, 3-4 minutes. Include garlic and seasonings; cook brief longer. Move to a 5-qt. slow cooker.

2.   In the same skillet, heat remaining oil over medium-high warmth. Include bulgur; cook and mix until daintily caramelized, 2-3 minutes or until softly sautéed.

3.   Include bulgur, tomatoes, stock, darker sugar, and soy sauce to slow cooker. Cook, secured, on low 3-4 hours or until bulgur is delicate. Mix in beans and raisins; cook 30 minutes longer.

Whenever wanted, sprinkle with cilantro.

Tofu Chow Mein

Total Time

Prep: 15 min. + standing Cook: 15 min.

Makes

4 servings

Ingredients:

- 8 ounces uncooked entire wheat holy messenger hair pasta
- 3 tablespoons sesame oil, separated
- 1 bundle (16 ounces) extra-firm tofu
- 2 cups cut new mushrooms
- 1 medium sweet red pepper, julienned
- 1/4 cup decreased sodium soy sauce
- 3 green onions daintily cut

Directions:

1.   Cook pasta as per bundle headings. Channel; flush with cold water and channel once more. Hurl with 1 tablespoon oil; spread onto a preparing sheet and let remain around 60 minutes.

2.   In the meantime, cut tofu into 1/2-in. 3D shapes and smudge dry. Enclose by a spotless kitchen towel; place on a plate and refrigerate until prepared to cook.

3.   In an enormous skillet, heat 1 tablespoon oil over medium warmth. Include pasta, spreading equitably; cook until base is daintily caramelized, around 5 minutes. Expel from skillet.

4.   In the same skillet, heat remaining oil over medium-high warmth; pan sear mushrooms, pepper, and tofu until mushrooms are delicate, 3-4 minutes. Include pasta and soy sauce; hurl and warmth through. Sprinkle with green onions.

Bow Ties with Sausage & Asparagus

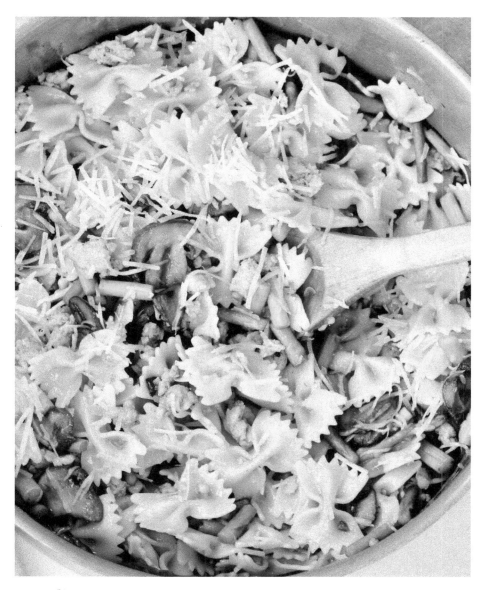

Ingredients

- 3 cups of uncooked whole wheat bow tie pasta (about 8 ounces)

- 1 pound of asparagus, cut into 1-1/2-inch pieces

- One package (19-1/2 ounces) Italian turkey sausage links, casings removed

- One medium onion, chopped

- Three garlic cloves, minced

- 1/4 cup shredded Parmesan cheese

- Additional shredded Parmesan cheese, optional

Instructions

1. In a 6-qt. Stockpot, prepare dinner pasta in line with package directions, including asparagus over the last 2-three minutes of cooking. Drain, reserving half cup pasta water; return pasta and asparagus to the pot.

2. Meanwhile, during a big skillet, cook sausage, onion and garlic over medium heat until no pink, 6-8 minutes, breaking sausage into large crumbles. increase stockpot. Stir in 1/four cup cheese and reserved pasta water as desired. Serve with additional cheese if desired.

Nutrition

247 calories, 7g fat (2g saturated fat), 36mg cholesterol, 441mg sodium, 28g carbohydrate (2g sugars, 4g fibre), 17g protein

Pork and Balsamic Strawberry Salad

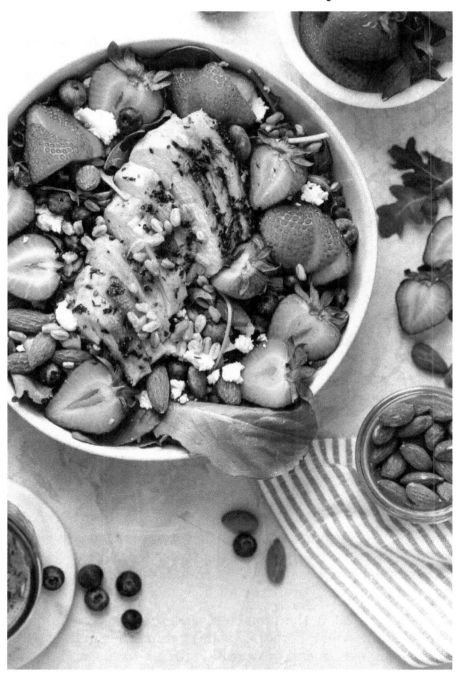

Ingredients

- One pork tenderloin (1 pound)
- 1/2 cup Italian salad dressing
- 1-1/2 cups halved fresh strawberries
- Two tablespoons balsamic vinegar
- Two teaspoons sugar
- 1/4 teaspoon salt
- 1/4 teaspoon pepper
- Two tablespoons olive oil
- 1/4 cup chicken broth

- One package about 5 ounces spring mix salad greens 1/2 cup crumbled goat cheese

Instructions

1.   Place pork during a shallow dish. Add salad dressing; flip for coating. Refrigerate and canopy for a minimum of eight hours. Mix strawberries, vinegar and sugar; cover and refrigerate.

2.   Preheat oven to 425°. Drain and wipe off meat , discarding marinade. Sprinkle with salt and pepper. during a large cast-iron or every other ovenproof skillet, warmness oil over medium-high warmness. Add beef; brown on all sides.

3.   Bake until a thermometer reads 145°, 15-20 minutes. Remove from skillet; permit or stand 5 min. Then, add broth to skillet; cook over medium warmth, stirring to loosen browned

bits from pan. bring back a boil. Reduce warmth; add strawberry. Then heat it.

4.   Place green vegetables on a serving platter; sprinkle with cheese. Slice pork; found out over veggies. Top with strawberry mixture.

Nutrition

291 calories, 16g fat (5g saturated fat), 81mg cholesterol, 444mg sodium, 12g carbohydrate (7g sugars, 3g fibre), 26g protein.

Peppered Tuna Kabobs

Ingredients

- 1/2 cup frozen corn, thawed Four green onions, chopped
- One jalapeno pepper, seeded and chopped
- Two tablespoons coarsely chopped fresh parsley
- Two tablespoons lime juice
- 1 pound tuna steaks, cut into 1-inch cubes
- One teaspoon coarsely ground pepper
- Two large sweet red peppers, cut into 2x1-inch pieces

Instructions

1.   One medium mango, peeled and cut into 1-inch cubes

2.   For salsa, during a small bowl, combine the primary five ingredients; put aside .

3.   Rub tuna with pepper. On 4metal or soaked wooden skewers, alternately thread red peppers, tuna and mango.

4.   Place skewers on greased grill rack. Cook, covered, over medium heat, occasionally turning, until tuna is slightly pink in centre

(medium-rare) and peppers are tender 10-12 minutes. Serve with salsa.

Nutrition

205 calories, 2g fat (0 saturated fat), 51mg cholesterol, 50mg sodium, 20g carbohydrate (12g sugars, 4g fibre), 29g protein.

Weeknight Chicken Chop Suey

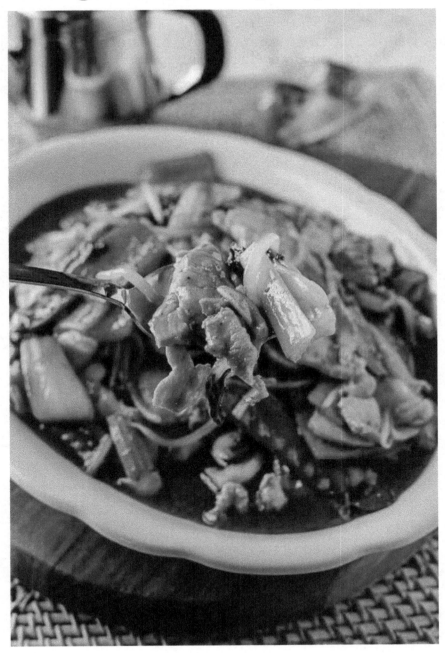

Ingredients

- Four teaspoons of olive oil

- 1 pound of boneless chicken breast side, cut into 1-inch cubes

- 1/2 teaspoon dried tarragon

- 1/2 teaspoon dried basil

- 1/2 teaspoon dried marjoram

- 1/2 teaspoon grated lemon zest

- 1-1/2 cups chopped carrots

- 1 cup unsweetened pineapple tidbits, drained (reserve juice)

- One can (8 ounces) sliced water chestnuts, drained

- One medium tart apple, chopped

- 1/2 cup chopped onion

- 1 cup cold water, divided

- Three tablespoons unsweetened pineapple juice

- Three tablespoons reduced-sodium teriyaki sauce

- Two tablespoons cornstarch

- 3 cups hot cooked brown rice

Instructions

1.   In a massive cast-iron or another heavy skillet, heat oil at medium temperature. Add chicken, herbs and lemon zest; leave

it until lightly browned. Add subsequent five ingredients. Stir in 3/four cup water, fruit juice and teriyaki sauce; bring back a boil. Reduce warmness; simmer covered till chicken is not any longer purple, and therefore the carrots are gentle 10-15 minutes.

2.   Combine cornstarch and remaining water. Gradually stir into hen mixture. Leave for boiling; cook and stir till thickened, about 2 minutes. Serve with rice.

Nutrition

330 calories, 6g fat, 42mg cholesterol, 227mg sodium, 50g carbohydrate (14g sugars, 5g fibre), 20g protein

Cucumber and Zucchini Soup

Serving: 3

Prep Time: 10 minutes + Chill time

Cook Time: nil

Ingredients:

- 2 tablespoons olive oil
- 1 tablespoon fresh dill
- 2/5 cup fresh cream
- 7 ounces cucumber, cubed
- 10 ½ zucchini, cubed
- 1 red pepper, chopped
- 3 celery stalks, chopped
- Sunflower seeds and pepper to taste

How To:

1. Add all the veggies during a juice and make a smooth juice.

2. Mix within the fresh cream and vegetable oil .

3.   Season with pepper and sunflower seeds.

4.   Garnish with dill.

5.   Serve chilled and enjoy!

Nutrition (Per Serving)

Calories: 100

Fat: 8g

Carbohydrates: 4g

Protein: 2g

Crockpot Pumpkin Soup

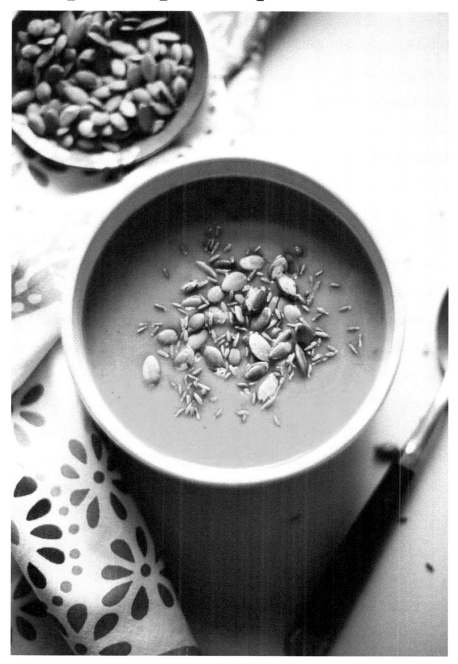

Serving: 3

Prep Time: 10 minute

Cook Time: 6-8 hours

Ingredients:

- 1 small pumpkin, halved, peeled, seeds removed, and pulp cubed
- 2 cups chicken broth
- 1 cup of coconut almond milk
- Sunflower seeds, pepper, thyme, and pepper, to taste

How To:

1. Add all the ingredients to a crockpot.

2. Close the lid.
3. Cook for 6-8 hours on LOW.
4. Make a smooth puree by employing a blender.
5. Garnish with roasted seeds.
6. Serve and enjoy!

Nutrition (Per Serving)

Calories: 60

Fat: 5g

Carbohydrates: 4g

Protein: 4g

Lightning Source UK Ltd.
Milton Keynes UK
UKHW020704130521
383649UK00005B/108